José Luís Esquijarosa Menéndez
Judiet González Díaz
Nielsen Bonilla Hernández

Antimicrobial susceptibility and resistance in infants with infections.

José Luís Esquijarosa Menéndez
Judiet González Díaz
Nielsen Bonilla Hernández

Antimicrobial susceptibility and resistance in infants with infections.

Pediatrics

Imprint

Any brand names and product names mentioned in this book are subject to trademark, brand or patent protection and are trademarks or registered trademarks of their respective holders. The use of brand names, product names, common names, trade names, product descriptions etc. even without a particular marking in this work is in no way to be construed to mean that such names may be regarded as unrestricted in respect of trademark and brand protection legislation and could thus be used by anyone.

Cover image: www.ingimage.com

This book is a translation from the original published under ISBN 978-620-2-16679-9.

Publisher:
Sciencia Scripts
is a trademark of
Dodo Books Indian Ocean Ltd. and OmniScriptum S.R.L publishing group

120 High Road, East Finchley, London, N2 9ED, United Kingdom
Str. Armeneasca 28/1, office 1, Chisinau MD-2012, Republic of Moldova, Europe
Printed at: see last page
ISBN: 978-620-7-88762-0

DEDICATION

*To my parents, thank you for your example, both professionally and personally.
Thank you for instilling in me the values and tools that have allowed me to get to
where I am today.*
To the children, who are our raison d'être.

ACKNOWLEDGEMENTS

To my parents, for their availability, support at all times and for their great affection and trust.

To my thesis tutor, Dr. Judiet González Díaz, and my advisor, Dr. Nielsen Bonilla Hernández, because with their teaching and patience, they have introduced me to the world of research.

To my family, friends and all the people who directly or indirectly have always given me their support.

I thank my dear teachers and colleagues, for without them I would not have been able to progress.

SUMMARY

A descriptive, longitudinal and prospective study was conducted at the Hospital Comandante Pinares in San Cristóbal, Artemisa province, during the period from May 2017 to May 2019 with the aim of determining the behaviour of antimicrobial susceptibility to first choice antimicrobials in infants with urinary tract infection. The variables studied were: age groups, sex, clinical forms of presentation, isolated germs, antimicrobial susceptibility and alterations in complementary examinations. The study universe consisted of 127 infants admitted to the paediatric ward with a diagnosis of urinary tract infection, respecting the inclusion and exclusion criteria. We observed that 3rd generation cephalosporins showed high levels of resistance while Amikacin showed a low level and the highest sensitivity was shown by Nitrofurantoin. Urinary tract infection predominated in females, except in the 1-3 months age group, where males predominated, with the highest incidence also in this age group. Escherichia coli was the most frequent cause of urinary tract infection, predominating in both sexes. The most frequent clinical forms of presentation were the dystrophic form, followed by the febrile and typical forms. A predominance of patients with leukocytosis and leukocyturia was observed.

Keywords: Urinary tract infection, infants, antimicrobial susceptibility.

TABLE OF CONTENTS

INTRODUCTION

Urinary tract infection (UTI) is a common pathology in childhood and one of the most common causes of paediatric emergency department visits. Clinical manifestations may be non-specific in infants and young children; however, in older children the symptomatology is more specific. It is one of the most common non-epidemic bacterial infections diagnosed in children worldwide, and is recognised as the third most common cause of infection after respiratory and diarrhoeal infections (1).

The accurate diagnosis and appropriate treatment of UTI is especially important to prevent renal damage. It most frequently affects female patients at all ages, with the exception of the first 3 months of life, when it predominates in males, generally associated with underlying congenital anomalies of the urinary tract. Approximately 3-5% of females and 1-2% of males have at least one episode of urinary tract infection during childhood. Several studies have reported a higher prevalence of UTI in Asians, followed by white and Hispanic children, and finally in African Americans (1, 2). (1, 2)

Some consider it a social disease because of its incidence, duration and possible sequelae. It is the most frequent cause of fever without focus in children under three years of age and is the most frequent nephrourological pathology encountered by the primary care paediatrician. The prevalence of urinary tract infection in febrile patients is 2.5% in boys and 8.8% in girls. It is also a parenteral cause of digestive disorders (diarrhoea and dehydration) or chronic nutritional disorders (malnutrition in infants) (3, 4, 5). (3, 4, 5).

Based on recent prospective studies, we can say that it is the most frequent bacterial infection in the paediatric age group, with a preferential incidence during the breastfeeding period. It is therefore a pathology that generates high morbidity during the acute phase with repeated visits to the paediatrician, requiring one or more rounds of antibiotic treatment and requiring hospitalisation on multiple occasions (3).

Their initial treatment is often empirical, so the choice of antimicrobial is based on epidemiology and local susceptibility patterns. The introduction of antibiotics into clinical practice was one of the most important interventions for the control of infectious diseases. Antibiotics have They have saved millions of lives, and have also revolutionised medicine. In the hospital setting, they are a highly prescribed therapeutic group and their misuse has generated major healthcare problems. In this sense, the assessment of the quality of prescribing allows managers and professionals to guide them towards the effective and safe use of these drugs and to detect areas for improvement, which implies knowledge about the prescription of the drug and the existence of a consensus for that indication. Prescribing-indication assessment is the best way to measure the use of medicines and is the most widely accepted by practitioners. (6, 7)

Unnecessary use of antimicrobials has clear undesirable effects for the patient (eradication of normal flora, increase and selection of resistant strains) and the community (modification of microbial susceptibility patterns and health expenditure); it can also lead to increased bacterial resistance. The ecology of resistance is a fairly young field and the real "puzzle" of the origin and evolution of bacterial resistance is still being investigated. According to data from the World Health Organisation, this is one of the major health problems worldwide (8, 9).

The modern era of antimicrobial therapeutics began in 1934 with Dogmak's description of the effectiveness of the first sulphonamide in the treatment of experimental streptococcal infections, the so-called "Golden Age" of antibiotics began in 1941 with the large-scale production of penicillin and its successful use in clinical trials, but today its widespread use is fuelling the rise of germ resistance, creating an increasing need for new drugs, and making treatment more expensive. Bacterial resistance to antibiotics is a global health problem that is constantly evolving. (10)

From a practical point of view, a bacterium is sensitive to an antibiotic when the antibiotic is effective against it and can be expected to cure the infection; on the other hand, it is resistant when its growth can only be inhibited at concentrations higher than the drug can reach at the site of infection. The emergence and spread of bacterial resistance is currently considered to be a growing phenomenon around the world and of great complexity (11).

New mechanisms of bacterial resistance to antibiotics are frequently reported in both gram-negative and gram-positive bacteria. The presence of Resistance in an infection-causing bacterium decreases the chances of clinical cure and bacteriological eradication and increases treatment costs, morbidity and mortality; therefore, it is important to select the appropriate treatment. Improving decisions on antimicrobial use ultimately requires guidance on treatment decisions made by patients and healthcare providers (12, 13).

Recently, the WHO published its first list of antibiotic-resistant "priority pathogens", which includes the twelve families of bacteria most dangerous to human health. The list was developed to try to guide and promote research and development of new antibiotics as part of efforts to combat the growing global problem. The list particularly highlights the threat posed by gram-negative bacteria resistant to multiple antibiotics. These bacteria have the innate ability to find new ways to resist treatment and can pass on genetic material that allows other bacteria to become drug-resistant. (14, 15) Currently, urinary tract infection is a worldwide problem. The overall prevalence in the paediatric population in Spain has been estimated at 5%, with an annual incidence of 3.1/1000 girls (0-14 years) and 1.7/1000 boys (0-14 years). In Chile, the overall incidence rate is 4.0/1,000 in children under 15 years of age, more frequent in males among children under one year of age, and predominantly in females among older children, similar to data from other countries. (3, 4)

During the first year of life, the incidence rate in the United States is 0.3-1.2 %, being more frequent in boys during the first three months of life, after this age it predominates in the female sex; in this country, between 2.4 and 2.8 % of children suffer from it each year; it causes more than 1.1 million paediatric consultations and generates a cost, exclusively due to hospital admissions for acute pyelonephritis, of more than 180 million dollars annually (3, 4).

Recent follow-up studies carried out in Sweden on a cohort of 1221 children with UTI have shown that 16-26 years after UTI, the risk of developing CKD is very low and limited exclusively to those with renal scarring in both kidneys. The same could be demonstrated for the development of high blood pressure (HBP), which was present in 9% of the children who developed scarring. compared to 6 % of those who suffered UTIs exclusively. In Mexico, in a series published by De la Cruz J. P. et al. of 100 children with UTIs demonstrated by suprapubic bladder puncture, predisposing urinary tract factors were found in 61 children, with vesicoureteral reflux being the most frequent (16).

In Cuba, a study carried out in the Nephrology Service of the "William Soler" Hospital in Havana reported an incidence of the disease of 1.4%; however, there are no population-based studies that show the incidence of this condition in the country. In a study conducted at the "Centro de Referencia de Nefrología Pediátrica de Cuba", three variables were found to be significantly associated with the development of renal scarring: vesicoureteral reflux, recurrence of UTI and age under five years (17).

SUBSTANTIATION OF THE SCIENTIFIC PROBLEM

One of today's major health problems is related to antibiotic resistance in several groups of bacteria, which has led the World Health Organisation (WHO) to ask the scientific community to find solutions to curb this problem, which has serious consequences for the world's population. Bacterial infections will cause more deaths from antibiotic resistance than cancer by 2050, making it the leading cause of death from disease in the world. The antimicrobial sensitivity of infection-causing bacteria is a dynamic development process, changing over time and with the frequent use of antibiotics, most of which are used indiscriminately, either by prescription or self-medication. (18, 19, 20)

Bacterial resistance to antibiotics is related to the consumption of antibiotics, favours the creation, adaptation and dissemination of antimicrobial resistance mechanisms whose increasing prevalence makes it essential to rationally guide the empirical treatment of urinary tract infection, which is a common and recommended practice. The resistance of pathogens to antimicrobial agents is a problem of extreme importance for the selection of the ideal first-line antibiotic, showing variations and requiring constant updating, microbiological surveillance of the antibiotic sensitivity of the main uropathogens that affect our environment. Because of the importance of Escherichia coli in the development of UTI and in other organs and systems, and the serious complications and sequelae that may occur as a result, it is necessary to conduct more extensive and continuous studies on the behaviour of antimicrobial susceptibility, as well as research that applies molecular biology to determine the mechanisms of resistance (21).

If the current trend persists, it could lead to a serious situation where relatively cheap and easy-to-administer oral antibiotics are no longer of practical benefit to young patients with UTIs. The result would be an increased reliance on much more expensive intravenous drugs. Considering the high number of patients presenting to our practices with urinary tract symptomatology and the vast majority with recurrences despite antibiotic management, we set out to conduct the study to update the prevalence of urinary tract infection in young patients with UTI and susceptibility to the antimicrobials used in empirical treatment (22).

Contextualisation of the behaviour of antimicrobial sensitivity and resistance to drugs of choice in urinary tract infection in the region of Artemisa province.

PRACTICAL INPUT

In each institution, service or ward, it is necessary to identify the main microorganisms that cause infectious processes, as well as their antimicrobial resistance pattern. This activity requires constant updating, thus becoming a research problem, which is addressed in the study that generates this research report. The study of urinary tract infection is of constant motivation for health professionals related to these patients, with the aim of improving the quality of care for children.

DEFINITION OF THE SCIENTIFIC PROBLEM

Scientific Problem.

What is the behaviour of antimicrobial sensitivity and resistance to drugs of first choice in infants with urinary tract infection admitted to the Paediatric Department of the "Comandante Pinares" Hospital?

SCIENTIFIC OBJECT OF RESEARCH.

The determination of the behaviour of antimicrobial susceptibility to drugs of first choice in infants (29 days old to 11 months and 29 days old) with urinary tract infection, attended in the Paediatrics service of the "Comandante Pinares" hospital in San Cristóbal from May 2017 to May 2019, including age groups, sex, clinical forms of presentation, isolated germs, antimicrobial susceptibility and alterations in complementary examinations.

REASONS JUSTIFYING THE PARTIES' PARTICIPATION.

In support of the World Health Organisation's strategy to contain antimicrobial resistance, it is the utmost responsibility of all health personnel to continue to join efforts aimed at the application of antimicrobial therapeutic policies that are always backed by the best scientific evidence. It is also the responsibility of all those of us directly involved in medical education to educate future physicians from a very early stage on the importance of appropriate antimicrobial prescribing and use, and to encourage them to teach their patients the importance of appropriate use of antimicrobials and the need to adhere to prescribed treatments. As a primary resource, work on disease prevention and infection control should continue.

THEORETICAL FRAMEWORK

Definition.

Urinary tract infection (UTI) is defined as the colonisation, invasion and multiplication in the urinary tract of pathogenic microorganisms, especially bacteria that usually come from the perineal region and overcome the host's defence mechanisms, producing an inflammatory reaction and morphological and functional alterations, with a clinical response that affects people of one sex or the other and different population groups with greater or lesser frequency. From a clinical point of view, it is difficult to establish a topographical diagnosis, mainly in younger children because the symptoms are very non-specific. However, clinical presentation can be defined according to location, evolution, structural involvement and recurrence. Operationally, urinary tract infection is defined as the coexistence of bacteriuria, leukocyturia and a significant number of bacteria in a urine culture (23).

Defence mechanisms of the urinary tract.

With the exception of the urethral mucosa, the urinary tract is generally resistant to bacterial colonisation because of the innate system response in the urinary tract. There is a strong proinflammatory response, and systemic production of interleukin 1□ and IL-6 can lead to activation of the acute phase response and fever. The severity of infection can be determined by serum and urine IL-6 concentration, with the highest levels observed in pyelonephritis and bacteraemia. On the other hand, the chemotactic cytokine IL-8 is released in the mucosa attracting polymorphonuclears (PMN), resulting in pyuria, which contributes to eradication of the condition. Infection stimulates the expression of CXCR1 and CXCR2 by urothelial cells; the former is essential for increasing neutrophil migration through infected cell layers in vitro. Urine is considered a good culture medium for most bacteria, although it has good antibacterial activity (24).

Anaerobic bacteria and other microorganisms make up the majority of the urethral microbiota, which do not usually multiply in urine. Similarly, extreme values of osmolarity, high urea concentration and low pH levels have been shown to inhibit the growth of some of the bacteria that cause UTI. The pH and The urine osmolarity of pregnant women tends to be more suitable for bacterial growth than that of non-pregnant women. The presence of glucose makes urine a better culture medium, while the addition of prostatic fluid to urine inhibits bacterial growth. Furthermore, urine has been shown to inhibit the migration, adherence, aggregation and elimination functions of PMNs (24).

Epidemiology.

The actual incidence and prevalence of UTIs varies with age, sex and diagnostic criteria, as well as the characteristics of the population studied. The cumulative risk for UTI during childhood is estimated to be 3-5% for girls and about 1% for boys. However, there is a higher incidence of UTI in newborns and male infants under one year of age, which is due to a higher frequency of obstructive anomalies of the lower urinary tract identified in this group of patients, such as urethral strictures and posterior urethral valve. After this age, it occurs more frequently in females due to various characteristics that favour it: anatomical proximity between the genitalia and the anus, short urethra and poor toilet technique.

Designations: (5)

1- Pyeloephritis: the renal parenchyma and pyelocaliceal system are affected.
2- Cystitis: limited to bladder.
3- Complicated UTI: anatomical or functional alterations or associated diseases.
4- Asymptomatic bacteriuria: presence of bacteria in urine culture without clinical symptoms.
5- Uncomplicated UTI: infections without structural alterations and good bladder emptying.
6- Recurrent UTI:
-Relapse: infection with the same germ after treatment has ended.
-Reinfection: another germ reappears after treatment.

7- Persistent UTI: persists during and after treatment.
There are 3 factors to consider in urinary tract infection, which are as follows: (25)
-Pathways of infection.

-Virulence factors: determined by the ability of the bacterium to colonise the urinary tract, cause disease and perpetuate itself. These factors have been attributed to different structures and properties of the bacteria.

-Host defence mechanisms: there are mechanisms that fight to prevent UTI by destroying the germ, when the virulence factors of the bacteria overcome the host defence mechanisms, UTI occurs.

Routes of infection. Microorganisms reach the kidney via ascending canalicular and haematogenous routes. Most gram-negative germs reach the urinary tract via the ascending route after colonisation of the perineal region and vaginal introitus in females or the subpreputial sac in males. The haematogenous route occurs mainly in the newborn, is the main route at this age and is observed when systemic sepsis occurs. For infection by the ascending canicular route to occur, it is necessary for the microorganisms to multiply to a large extent, which allows them to multiply:

–Colonise the vulvar region or the subpreputial sac.

–Ascend the urethra, reach the bladder and multiply.

–Resist the dragging mechanism exerted by urination.

Virulence factors. They are attributed to different properties of the bacteria that favour these factors:

–Presence of fimbriae (adherence):

• Fimbriae type I.

• Fimbrias type II or P.

• Adhesins X, M and S.

–Production of haemolysin, urease and colicin.

–Resistance to the bactericidal action of serum.

–Aerobactin system.

–O, K and H antigens.

–Bacterial resistance.

Host response. These include:

– Urinary pH: acidic pH prevents bacterial growth.

– Urinary osmolarity: between 350 and 1 200 stimulates bacterial growth.

– Bladder emptying: correct emptying prevents residual urine that would be a breeding ground.

– Presence of mucin: the bladder produces mucin that prevents bacterial adherence.

– Tamm Horsfall protein: binds to type I fimbriae in the bladder and both are excreted in the urine.

– Secretion of immunoglobulins: these have a bactericidal action.

– Inflammatory response: interleukins, tumour necrosis factor (TNF), interferon, nuclear polymorphs, macrophages, vasoactive substances and oxygen free radicals are released.

– Immune response: cellular or humoral.

Aetiology.

As part of the aetiology of this entity, it is noted that most urinary pathogens are part of the normal intestinal microbiota and have virulence factors that allow them to colonise the perineum in women and the foreskin in men, and then ascend to the bladder and kidney (4). In the neonatal period or in specific circumstances, infection may occur via the haematogenous route and on other occasions there may be infection via the lymphatic route. The literature describes the main uropathogenic agents of UTI as being Gram of intestinal origin. The most frequently encountered microorganism is Escherichia coli (86-90%), the rest being distributed mostly among Klebsiella spp, Proteus mirabilis, Enterobacter spp, Enterococcus spp, and Pseudomonas spp, the latter generally originating from nosocomial infections in immunocompromised patients, associated with congenital malformations of the urinary tract and urological instrumentation among other predisposing factors. Other microorganisms such as yeasts, viruses, protozoa and parasites cause UTIs less frequently (25).

Predisposing factors.

The presence of anatomical factors such as malformations, which cause stasis and obstruction, also increase the predisposition to infections, including vesicoureteral reflux, posterior urethral valvula and vulvar synechia, whose prevalence in paediatrics is 1.8%, frequently occurring between 3 months and 6 years of age. Urinary flow obstruction may predispose to postvoid dribbling, dysuria and urinary tract infection (UTI). (26)These factors, in turn, are classified as organic and functional (neurogenic bladder). Predisposing factors: (25)

–Poor grooming technique.

–Urinary tract obstruction.

–Calculations.

–Vesicoureteral reflux.

–Congenital anomalies of the bladder and urethra.

–Neurological bladder abnormalities.

–Renal trauma.

–Pregnancy.

Among the predisposing factors, grooming techniques become predictable factors: girls are not bathed.

Clinical picture.

Clinical manifestations are influenced by age, sex, presence or absence of predisposing factors, location of infection, interval of last infection (4).

Newborn: In the newborn, symptoms are non-specific and indistinguishable from other symptoms of infection in other locations. Hypothermia, fever, cyanosis, generalised sepsis, refusal of food, convulsions, vomiting (26).

Infant and transitional: the clinical picture is also non-specific, presenting in different ways: (4, 27)

-Dystrophic or cachectising: stationary weight as the only symptom.

-Acute febrile syndrome: fever without focus, without other accompanying symptoms.

-Sepsis: with systemic inflammatory response syndrome.

-Asymptomatic bacteriuria: presence of bacteria in a sample collected without presenting any symptoms.

Toxic-infectious: confined to renal abscess.

-Gastroenteric: presence of gastrointestinal symptoms of diarrhoea and vomiting, the latter predominating.

-Pseudomeningeal: characterised by bulging fontanel and irritability that can be mistaken for meningeal symptoms.

-Low symptomatology. Dysuria, pollakiuria.

Older child: Among children >2 years, most symptoms are referred to the urinary system and abdomen, making it easier to make a diagnosis of suspicion. When these symptoms are present, whether or not accompanied by fever, a general urine examination is recommended. The characteristic clinical features of urinary tract infection are observed depending on the anatomical location. In upper urinary tract infections (pyelonephritis), fever, chills, dysuria, lumbago, vomiting, abdominal pain appear. When the urinary tract infection is located at the bladder level (lower urinary tract infection), the clinical picture consists of dysuria, pollakiuria, urinary urgency, abdominal pain and often the urine has a haematuric appearance, with the absence of fever and symptoms of general involvement being characteristic of this clinical form. (25)

Diagnosis.

It is currently accepted that all UTIs should be confirmed by urine culture which in microbiological terms would be established by the number of colony forming units per millilitre of urine (cfu/mL). Accepted values are a colony count greater than 100 000 cfu/mL if the sample is collected by collection bag or midstream in a symptomatic child, greater than 10 000 cfu/mL if obtained by bladder catheterisation or any count if the urine sample is collected by bladder puncture. It should be assessed on a case-by-case basis and a systematic approach should be adopted for each paediatric case. The three basic aspects to consider are: (28)
–Assess the clinical symptoms and the patient's age: high or low UTI symptoms and age older or younger than 2-3 years.
–Assess simple biological methods of UTI topography: C-reactive protein, ESR, leukocytes, etc.
–Assess the urinary tract by performing an ultrasound scan in the acute phase (at diagnosis). Renal and urinary tract ultrasound should be performed in all children with a first episode of UTI because up to 12% of morphological abnormalities may be found (29).
Depending on the results of these assessments, the paediatrician will be able to classify the urinary tract infection in each specific case as a UTI with a low or high risk of kidney damage:
–Low-risk urinary tract infection: this is when the child is older than 3 to 5 years and has a normal ultrasound scan. The clinical symptomatology will be lower tract (dysuria, pollakiuria, etc.) and the biological signs of localisation will be normal.

–High-risk urinary tract infection: this is when the child is less than 2-3 years of age, or when the ultrasound is abnormal regardless of age, or when the child has symptoms of high UTI (fever, general condition, back pain, etc.) and/or the biological signs of localisation are positive.

Management of the child with low-risk UTI and choice of antibiotic treatment:
In low-risk UTIs, oral antibiotic treatment is recommended for a period of 7 days. Recommended antibiotics include ampicillin- augmentin, Nitrofurantoin, nalidixic acid and sulfamethoxazole-trimethoprim. In children >2 years: The most commonly used alternatives are:
-Trimethoprim-sulfamethoxazole at a dose of 50 mg/kg/day in 2 doses for 7 to 10 days.
-Ciprofloxacin at a dose of 15 mg/kg/day in 2 doses for 7 to 10 days.
-Cephalexin at a dose of 50 mg/kg/day in 3 doses for 7 to 10 days.
In all cases, a new culture should be taken 2 days after the end of treatment. Other antibiotic alternatives are:
-Cefuroxime-axetil, 15-20 mg/kg/day in 2 doses, for 5 days (especially indicated in at-risk patients such as uropaths, given the high sensitivity of the usual germs, >90%).

-Cefixime 8 mg/kg/day in 2 doses for 5 days.
-Cefaclor 30 mg/kg/day in 3 doses for 5 days.
In all cases, the efficacy of the treatment should be verified with a new urine culture three days after the treatment has started and one three to four days after the end of the treatment. If the urine culture result is negative, the child may be discharged. If the urine culture results are positive or if the infection recurs, the child should be managed as a high-risk UTI.

Management of the child with high-risk UTI and choice of treatment:

Antibiotic treatment shall be administered as early as possible, intravenously, preferably in the hospital environment and for a period of 7-14 days. A urine culture should be checked three and fifteen days after starting antibiotic treatment, and after three to six weeks a CURM should be performed after a negative urine culture in cases of recurrence. The antibiotics of choice include aminoglycosides (Amikacin), third generation cephalosporins (Cefotaxime, Ceftriaxone), etc. In high-risk UTI, the patient will be hospitalised and antibiotic therapy with Ceftriaxone 100 mg/kg/day in two doses will be started as first-line treatment. Subsequent management: once treatment has been completed and cure has been verified, an examination (renal US and DMSA and cystography if appropriate) and outpatient follow-up should be carried out in the following cases: (30,31)

a.- High-risk infection. b.- Age less than 5 years.

c.- More than two ITUs, even if they have been casualties.

d.- Suspected or confirmed cases of obstructive uropathies

Long-term prophylaxis is indicated in patients at risk of developing renal scarring, often caused by vesicoureteral reflux (VUR) and recurrent UTIs. It is used for reflux until it disappears and for recurrent UTIs for 6 to 12 months. Antibiotics that cause bacterial resistance in the gut should not be used. They are used in a single dose:

• Nitrofurantoin: 1-2 mg/kg/day

-Cotrimoxazole:10 mg/kg/day

• Nalidixic acid: 15-20 mg/kg/day

• Cephalexin:10 mg/kg/day

*Chemoprophylaxis is used at 9pm.

There are controversies in the treatment of UTI, due to the risk of encountering resistant strains, the delay in laboratory results, and the patient's need for prompt treatment. Despite the wide coverage of existing antibiotics to treat UTI, sometimes the urinary symptoms do not disappear due to risk factors or even more so due to a growing phenomenon of concern to the national and international medical community called bacterial resistance.More than half a century after the discovery of antibiotics, infections and infectious diseases remain the major cause of morbidity and mortality today. Rapid treatment with antimicrobials can mean the difference between cure and death or chronic disability for the infected patient. (10,32)

Unnecessary use of antimicrobials has clear undesirable effects for the patient (eradication of normal flora, increase and selection of resistant strains) and the community (modification of microbial susceptibility patterns and health care costs), and may lead to increased bacterial resistance. According to data from the World Health Organisation, bacteria have demonstrated a remarkable capacity to develop resistance, and have become a major problem worldwide (11,13, 33, 34).Latin America has the highest rates of antimicrobial resistance compared to some regions in the United States and Europe, which report carbapenem resistance rates of 25%, except in Greece, with 51%. Several studies indicate that Pseudomonas aeruginosa represents the fourth most common multidrug-resistant microorganism isolated from the intensive care unit, followed by E. coli, S. aureus and Klebsiella pneumoniae. Drug resistance occurs when micro-organisms, whether bacteria, viruses, fungi or parasites, undergo changes that render the drugs used to cure infections caused by them ineffective. Microorganisms that are resistant to most antimicrobials are known as ultra-resistant (35, 36, 37, 38, 39).

The high resistance to antimicrobials described above is probably related to their frequent use, ease of acquisition, low cost and the length of time they have been circulating in the community. However, recent research highlights how DNA from a bacterial cell in the environment can be transferred from one cell to another by one of the mechanisms of gene transfer. This, coupled with analytical studies Phylogenetic studies currently underway have provided insight into the evolution of resistance genes and support the possible impact that the use of antibiotics in agriculture and animal fattening may also have on the phenomenon, practices that are widespread, strongly debated and the cause of multiple contradictions on an international scale. Moreover, as E. coli is part of the human flora, antimicrobial treatments for infections other than urinary tract infections - such as respiratory, skin, intestinal and other infections where such antimicrobials are used - lead to the emergence of resistance of this micro-organism. How does it occur and what mechanisms are involved in microbial resistance?

Bacterial resistance can be natural or intrinsic and acquired, and must be analysed from several perspectives (pharmacokinetics, pharmacodynamics, population, molecular and clinical). Natural or intrinsic resistance is a specific property of bacteria, its occurrence predates the use of antibiotics and has the characteristic of being inherent to a particular species. The acquisition of genetic material by antimicrobial-susceptible bacteria can occur by exchange of genetic material from other bacteria or phages (viruses that use bacteria for their development and reproduction), through mechanisms such as: (40, 41)

1. Transformation: Transfer or incorporation by a bacterium of free extracellular DNA from the lysis of other bacteria.

2. Transduction: Transfer of chromosomal or plasmid DNA from one bacterium to another by means of a bacteriophage (virus that infects bacteria).

3. Transposon: Movement of a section of DNA (transposon) that may contain genes

for resistance to different antibiotics and other cassette genes linked in a kit for expression of a particular promoter.

4. Conjugation: Exchange of genetic material between two bacteria (donor and recipient), through a sexual strand or physical contact between the two.

The use of antimicrobial agents also creates selective pressure for the emergence of resistant strains (42).

Resistance definitions are classified according to the number and class of antibiotics affected. Multiple Drug Resistance (MDR) is defined as the absence of susceptibility to at least one drug in three or more of the antibiotic categories; Extensively Drug-Resistant (XDR) refers to the absence of susceptibility to at least one agent in all but two or fewer antimicrobial categories; and resistance to all antimicrobials is defined as resistance to all antibiotic categories. (43)

Resistance mechanisms depend on the type of bacteria that develop them. The gram-positive bacteria that most frequently cause infections in humans and have therefore developed resistance mechanisms are mostly staphylococci, streptococci (including pneumococci) and enterococci. On the other hand, resistance mechanisms of Streptococcus pneumoniae strains, and of beta-haemolytic and viridans group streptococci stand out. Among the non-fermenting gram-negative bacilli, strains of Pseudomonas aeruginosa remain the main cause of bacteraemia, although infections by strains of Acinetobacter spp. are also proliferating (44).

The emergence of microorganisms producing extended-spectrum b-lactamases (ESBLs), capable of inactivating potent cephalosporins, has generated great concern due to the clinical and therapeutic implications they have, because they are transmitted by plasmids and can therefore spread to many microorganisms, the spread of resistance to extended-spectrum cephalosporins further limits the use of b-lactams and stimulates the use of more costly and broader-spectrum antibiotics; but, in addition, these resistant strains may go undetected by routine microbiological procedures and thus lead to frequent and sometimes fatal treatment failures. Extended-spectrum ß-lactamases are enzymes produced by Gram-negative bacilli, mainly enterobacteria such as Klebsiella pneumoniae and Escherichia coli, but also by non-fermenting microorganisms such as Pseudomonas aeruginosa and others (45).Nowadays, the existing microbial resistance, with multi-resistant and ultra-resistant germs, requires the improvement and better control of antimicrobial policies in each health institution. Antimicrobial Policy can be defined as: "A set of measures that have the primary purpose of tailoring antimicrobial therapy effectively to each patient, with a minimum of complications, avoid adverse reactions, control the possibility of the development and spread of resistant strains of micro-organisms, and reduce hospital costs as much as possible. It is the set of rules that regulate the use of antibiotics in a health care area or facility. It is an ongoing process of setting out criteria for the appropriate selection of antimicrobials (42).

The European Consensus on Antibiotic Use recommends: "Controlling the consumption of antimicrobial agents, instituting a selective list of antibiotics to be used in hospital treatment guidelines and limiting the introduction of new antibiotics without certain criteria on activity, toxicity, pharmacokinetics and cost" (46, 47). (46, 47)Since 1996, Cuba has been a member of the Alliance for the Prudent Use of Antibiotics (APUA), an international organisation made up of more than 60 national chapters on five continents and with individual members from more than 100 countries. This organisation was created as a specialised professional response to promote the appropriate use of antimicrobials, to understand the problems arising from the use of these compounds in society, and to disseminate the principles of their rational use in communities affected by infectious diseases.(48)

AINIA (Spain) is investigating the application of bacteriophages as antibiotic substitutes. Bacteriophages, also called phages, are viruses that infect bacteria and are capable of killing the bacteria responsible for various diseases, thus representing a possible alternative to tackle the problem of antibiotic resistance. Moreover, unlike antibiotics, phages affect only the target bacterium without harming any other cells and no side effects have been described in their use (19).

OBJECTIVES

General.

To determine the behaviour of antimicrobial sensitivity and resistance to drugs of first choice in infants with urinary tract infection, in the Paediatric Department of the General Hospital "Comandante Pinares", during the period from May 2017 to May 2019.

Specific.

1- To distribute patients diagnosed with UTI according to age and sex.

2- To identify the most frequent uropathogenic germs in infants in our environment in relation to sex.

3- Determine the susceptibility of the isolated microorganisms to Ceftriaxone and Amikacin.

4- Determine the susceptibility of the isolated micro-organisms to second-line drugs.

5- To identify the most frequent clinical forms of presentation in infants in our environment.

6- To determine which complementary tests were most altered in the patients studied.

METHODOLOGICAL DESIGN

Type of study.

An analytical, longitudinal and prospective study was conducted in the Paediatric Department of the General Hospital "Comandante Pinares", San Cristóbal municipality, Artemisa, during the period from May 2017 to May 2019.

Universe.

The study universe consisted of 127 infants between 29 days of birth and 11 months and 29 days of age who were admitted to the Paediatric Department of the General Hospital "Comandante Pinares", in the municipality of San Cristóbal, Artemisa, with a diagnosis of urinary tract infection, who were included in their entirety in the study, as they fulfilled the required criteria.

Inclusion criteria.

-Patients aged between 29 days old and 11 months and 29 days admitted with a presumptive diagnosis of UTI.

With positive urine cultures: micro-organisms isolated from urine samples collected by midstream or spontaneous urination technique with a count greater than 100 000 cfu/mL, or by bladder catheterisation technique with a count greater than 10 000 cfu/mL, or by bladder puncture technique with any bacterial growth.

- That parents gave consent to participate in the research. Exclusion criteria.

-Patients under 29 days of age and over 11 months and 29 days of age.

-Negative or contaminated urine cultures according to the above criteria.

-Those whose parents did not agree to participate in the study.

INFORMATION GATHERING

Sources of information.

The necessary information was collected through a record sheet for each patient (Annex 2) with the data obtained from the review of individual medical records, the record book of positive urine cultures and antibiogram results from the Microbiology laboratory of the "Comandante Pinares" Hospital, which were updated periodically, allowing for uniformity in the clinical information. The information obtained was recorded in a Microsoft Excel database for initial verification and verification of the veracity of the data, avoiding duplications and errors, which was guaranteed by double reading of the data by two other research collaborators.

Information processing technique.

The information obtained was recorded in a Microsoft Access database and frequency distribution and contingency tables were drawn up where the absolute and relative frequency of qualitative variables were analysed and interpreted, as well as the chi-square statistical technique (X^2), for qualitative variables and the means, standard deviation and Student's t-test for independent samples for quantitative variables with a significance level of a = 0.05. The final report, tables and graphs were written using the text editor Word for Windows 10.

OPERATIONALISATION OF THE VARIABLES

A. The following variables were studied to address objective 1:

Variable	Type	Operationalisation		Indicator
		Scale	Description	
Groups Age groups	Quantitative Ordinal	29 days - 3 months 4- 6 months 7 - 9 months 10- 11 months and 29 days	The last month served shall be included	Number and percentage
Sex	Qualitative Nominal Dichotomous	Female Male	According to biological sex	Number and percentage

B. The following variables were studied to address objective 2:

Variable	Type	Operationalisation		Indicator
		Scale	Description	
Isolated germs	Qualitative Nominal Nominal Polytomous	Escherichia coli. Klebsiella spp. Proteus spp. Enterobacter spp. Citrobacter freundii. Others.	According to data collected in the book register of positive urine cultures. Gram-negative bacilli, no species identified.	Number and percentage

C. The following variables were studied to achieve objectives 3 and 4:

Variable	Type	Operationalisation		Indicator
		Scale	Description	
Antimicrobial susceptibility	Qualitative Nominal Dichotomous	Sensitive Resistant	According to data collected in the antibiogram results from the laboratory of the Microbiology	Antimicrobial Susceptibility

D. The following variables were studied to address objective 5:

Variable	Type	Operationalisation		Indicator
		Scale	Description	
Forms Presentation clinics	Qualitative Nominal Nominal Polytomous	Typical Asymptomatic Asymptomatic Febrile Dystrophic Dystrophic Methaemia Diarrhoeic Anaemic Icteric Pseudomeningeal Toxic Infectious	According to data collected in the medical records, by means of the interview with parents or guardians	Number and percentage

F. The following variables were studied to address objective 6:

Variable	Type	Operationalisation		Indicator
		Scale	Description	
		Anemia		
Alterationsin complementary examinations	Qualitative Nominal Nominal Polytomous	Leukocytosis Accelerated erythrocyte sedimentation rate Leucocyturia Ultrasonographic alterations	According to data collected in the medical records, by means of the interview with parents or guardians	Number and percentage

BIOETHICAL CONSIDERATIONS

Based on the application of the principles of bioethics, the principles of beneficence and non-maleficence were put into practice, as the research was risk-free and the information can be used at a later stage to reverse the negative aspects. During the collection of information there were no privileges, respecting the principle of justice, and taking into account compliance with the principles stipulated in the Nuremberg Code (1947) and the Declaration of Helsinki (2013), we requested explicit informed consent (Annex 1) from the patients, after having correctly informed them about what, why and for what purpose we are doing the study.

Table I: Infants with urinary tract infection. Distribution according to age and sex. General Teaching Hospital "Comandante Pinares". San Cristóbal. 2017- 2019.

MALE FEMALE TOTAL Age groups

	No.	%	No.	%	No.	%
1 - 3 months	26	20.5	25	19.7	51	40.2
4- 6	14	11.0	30	23.6	44	34.6
7 - 9	9	7.1	14	11.0	23	18.1
10- 11 months and 29 days	2	1.6	7	5.5	9	7.1
TOTAL	51	40.2	76	59.8	127	100.0
Media and Ds	4,2 ± 2,7		5,1 ± 2,8			

t = 1,8012p =0,0741

Source: Medical records.

Table I shows that there was a predominance of the female sex with 59.8 % over the male sex with 40.2 % in a 3:2 ratio, except in the ages between 1 and 3 months of age, where the male sex predominated with a total of 26 cases (20.5%) while the female sex was represented by 25 (19.7%), also in this age group there was a higher incidence of urinary tract infection with a total of 51 cases for 40.2 %. These results are consistent with those found in an extensive review of the world and national literature. The higher prevalence in the female sex implies a higher risk of UTI in girls, due to the proximity of the perianal area to the urinary meatus, the shortness of the urethra and poor toilet techniques. The higher incidence of UTI in newborns (1-4%) and male infants in the first 3 months is due to the higher prevalence of obstructive anomalies of the lower urinary tract, particularly identified in this age group. (49-52) In terms of age and sex, a study conducted in Madrid in 2010 found that in the first 3 months of life, infection is more frequent in males. A study conducted at the Hospital de San José, in the city of Bogotá, during the period from October 2015 to July 2016 showed a higher prevalence in girls, being more frequent in boys in the first 6 months of life, and then predominating in women, with a ratio of 10 to 1. In the Hospital Universitario de la ciudad de Guayaquil, in the period from June 2014 to June 2015, in relation to sex, there was a greater presence of urinary tract infection in girls. (3,

53, 54).The Laboratory of the National Secretariat for the Human Rights of Persons with Disabilities "Fernando de la Mora," in Paraguay, reports that of the samples studied, 10/21 (48%) were positive in boys and 11/21 (52%) in girls. Different results are reported in a publication by the Acta Pediátrica de México in January 2018 where in the first year of life it was more frequent in boys (3.7%) than in girls (2%). (55, 56)

An investigation carried out on patients treated at the Hospital "General Milanés" with a presumptive diagnosis of urinary sepsis, belonging to the Bayamo area during 1999 showed a difference by months of age in both sexes, with urosepsis predominating in boys up to 4 months and after 5 months - 1 year in girls (62% and 54.5%, respectively). This result is consistent with a study from the Paediatric Hospital of Guantánamo in 2007 (1).

In the microbiology laboratory of the "Juan Manuel Márquez" Paediatric Hospital, between 1 January and 31 December 2010, out of 579 positive urine culture samples, 420 (72.5 %) were female and 159 (27.5 %) were male. A study carried out in the municipality of Banes, Holguín, from November 2012 to October 2013, showed a predominance of the female sex (90 %) (21, 57). Similar results were obtained in the Provincial Microbiology Laboratory of Mayabeque, in the municipality of San José de las Lajas, in the period between May and December 2012, where 74.41 % of all positive urine cultures were in the female sex, with a ratio of 3:1, i.e. for every 4 females with positive urine cultures there was one male with a positive urine culture. (58)In another study carried out at the "Pedro Agustín Pérez" Paediatric Teaching Hospital in Guantánamo from January to December 2013, out of 384 patients studied, more than two thirds were in the first group (older than 29 days old to 6 months) with 267 infants for 69.5 % and only 117 were in the age group from 6 months and 1 day to 11 months and 29 days for 30.5 %. In both groups the female sex was predominant, 192 cases for 50 % in the first age group and 83 for 21.6 % in the second group (59).

Table II: Germs isolated from urine cultures. Distribution of identified uropathogens according to sex. General Teaching Hospital "Comandante Pinares". San Cristóbal. 2017- 2019.

Germs	Male		Female		Total	
	No.	%	No.	%	No.	%
Escherichia coli	21	16.5	39	30.7	60	47.2
Klebsiella spp.	3	2.4	5	3.9	8	6.3
Proteus spp.	10	7.9	7	5.5	17	13.4
Enterobacter spp.	8	6.3	10	7.9	18	14.2
Cytobacter freundii	3	2.4	6	4.7	9	7.1
Other	6	4.7	9	7.1	15	11.8
Total	51	40.2	76	59.8	127	100.0

$X^2 = 3,4646$ $p = 0.6287$

Source: Urine culture record book. Microbiology Laboratory. General Hospital Docent "Comandante Pinares."

Table II shows that, as in most UTI investigations, in our study Escherichia coli is recognised as the microorganism that most frequently constituted the cause of urinary tract infection, with a percentage of isolation of 47.2%, predominating in both sexes.2%, predominating in both sexes, followed by Enterobacter spp. (14.2%) and Proteus spp. (13.4%), which tripled in presentation; these results are similar to those published by national and international authors of studies on the prevalence of bacterial microorganisms in urine cultures performed in children. In general, the germs isolated predominated in the female sex, with the exception of Proteus, which was isolated in 10 male patients and 7 female patients. Proteus is the second most mobile gram-negative bacillus in the faecal flora, found in 30 % of male UTIs and very often colonising the foreskin. This result was to be expected considering that, internationally, E. coli is the uropathogen par excellence in both community and nosocomial infections. (4, 26)This is explained by two theories that emerged and were developed in the 1960s: the "Prevalence" and "Special Pathogenicity" theories. The first theory states that the micro-organism that is most abundant in the intestinal microbiota will be the one with the highest frequency in the intestinal microbiota. The second hypothesises that only a select group of strains with virulence factors cause infection. In the case of E. coli, this is the main agent found in the intestinal microbiota, and it has been demonstrated that it presents various virulence factors such as adhesins, K1 antigens and a-hemolysin, among others. When reviewing the medical literature on the subject, authors such as Goldraich NP et al. and Ronald A., in 2002, have pointed out the broad bacterial aetiology of UTI in children. In an investigation carried out in the microbiology laboratory belonging to the Municipal Centre of Hygiene and Epidemiology, in Güines, in the period from 2003 to 2004, showed that more than 95 % of "uncomplicated" UTI were caused by gram-negative bacilli and among them enterobacteria, of which Escherichia coli was the most frequent. In the study of the Microbiology laboratory of the Amalia Simoni Provincial University Hospital in the city of Camagüey, between January 2008 and December 2014, gram-negative bacteria prevailed (92.47 %), led by Escherichia coli, followed by Citrobacter freundii and Pantoea agglomerans, which quadrupled in presentation (60,61).Also in the "Juan Manuel Márquez" Paediatric Hospital in the period from 1 January to 31 December 2010, E. coli was the predominant microorganism in the urine culture records in both sexes. The other most frequently found microorganisms were Klebsiella spp, Proteus spp and Serratia spp, the latter being a bacterium of growing importance according to international literature, which causes urinary tract infection of nosocomial origin in children with urinary tract instrumentation; these isolation percentages are similar to those reported in other national investigations (1, 21, 49, 59, 62, 63).Our results are similar to a study carried out at the Hospital Universitario Central de Asturias (Oviedo, Asturias) between January 2009 and December 2013 in a paediatric population under 14 years of age, reporting that 81.4% of the isolates corresponded to three germs: Escherichia coli, Enterococcus ssp. and Proteus mirabilis, the former being the most frequently isolated microorganism (58.9% of the total number of positive urine cultures). Enterococcus ssp. and P. mirabilis followed E. coli in frequency, with 11.6% and 10.9%, respectively, of total isolates. Other less frequently isolated microorganisms were Kle- bsiella pneumoniae, Pseudomonas aeruginosa and Klebsiella oxytoca with 3.4%, 2.6% and 2.9%, respectively, of total isolates. 1.3% of cases, respectively, similar to data published in other studies (64, 65, 66, 67). In the University Hospital of the city of Guayaquil, in the period from June 2014 to June 2015, cultures were positive for 3 main causative agents, with E. coli topping the list with 24 cases, equivalent to 86 %, Proteus Mirabilis with 3 cases, equivalent to 11 %, and Klebsiella 3 % with 1 case. The Laboratory of the National Secretariat for the Human Rights of

Persons with Disabilities "Fernando de la Mora", Paraguay, reports that the most frequently isolated germ in their study was E. coli, 11/21 (52%), which correlates with other studies carried out by López Genaro et al (54, 55, 68).

Table III: Antimicrobial susceptibility. Distribution of drugs analysed according to sensitivity and resistance patterns. General Teaching Hospital "Comandante Pinares". San Cristóbal. 2017- 2019.

Antibiotic	Sensitivity		Resistance		Total n=127	
	No.	%	No.	%	No.	%
Ceftriaxone	19	15.0	108	85.0	127	100.0
Amikacin	92	72.4	35	27.6	127	100.0
Cefotaxime	32	25.2	95	74.8	127	100.0
Ciprofloxacin	69	54.3	58	45.7	127	100.0
Cotrimoxazole	67	52.8	60	47.2	127	100.0
Nalidixic acid	65	51.2	62	48.8	127	100.0
Nitrofurantoin	100	78.7	27	21.3	127	100.0
Cephalexin	52	40.9	75	59.1	127	100.0
Amoxicillin	17	13.4	110	86.6	127	100.0

Source: Urine culture record book. Microbiology Laboratory. General Hospital Docent "Comandante Pinares."

Urinary tract infection is common in paediatrics and once the diagnosis has been made, empirical treatment should be started, to be re-evaluated when the results of the culture and antibiogram are obtained or, in their absence, according to the clinical response. However, it is advisable, from time to time, to evaluate the sensitivity of the bacteria that cause this disease, as their ability to develop resistance to the antibiotics used is well known, hence the importance of this study. Recently, a new plasmid, New Delhi metallo-b-lactamases (NDM-1), was identified in E. coli, t h e E. coli strains producing these enzymes. are resistant to many groups of antibiotics, including fluoroquinolones, aminoglycosides, b-lactams and even carbapenemics (10). [ra]Table III analyses the levels of sensitivity and resistance identified in the uropathogens isolated in our study, with respect to the most commonly used antimicrobials in the treatment of urinary tract infections, paying special attention to the 3rd generation Cephalosporins (mainly Ceftriaxone) and Aminoglycosides (Amikacin), the first choice drugs protocolised in the treatment of high-risk UTI, a group that includes the patients selected for this study.

The highest levels of resistance were observed for Amoxicillin with 86.6%, followed by the 3-generation cephalosporins[ra], Ceftriaxone and Cefotaxime with 85.0% and 74.8% respectively. Resistance to these cephalosporins may be due to the presence of extended spectrum beta-lactamases (ESBL). This fact leads to the need to include phenotypic methods to detect their presence in antimicrobial susceptibility studies performed in hospitals. Similar studies reviewed show that the incidence of extended-spectrum beta-lactamases is increasing and that infections caused by BLEE-producing microorganisms are resistant to all penicillins, and also to third and fourth generation cephalosporins, which limits the therapeutic options (1).

Amikacin, on the other hand, showed a low level of resistance with 27.6%. We believe that this result is due to the low use of this drug, because despite being a drug of 1[ra] line of treatment, its use is controversial and limited due to its known nephrotoxic and ototoxic properties. The most important mechanism of resistance to aminoglycosides remains enzyme inactivation (22).

Nitrofurantoin showed the highest level of sensitivity with 78.7%. We believe that this is due to the low indication for this drug, due to the frequent gastrointestinal adverse reactions it causes, and to the fact that UTI treatment protocols always start with parenteral drugs. In addition, this drug is recommended for outpatient oral therapy in low infections, but not in high infections due to its low concentration in plasma and renal tissue.Average sensitivity patterns showed the antibiotics: Ciprofloxacin (54.3%), Cotrimoxazole (52.8%), Nalidixic acid (51.2%) and Cephalexin (40.9%). In recent years Several studies have shown a decrease in the sensitivity of E. coli to ciprofloxacin, and it is suggested that resistance may be due to chromosomal mutations and plasmid genes encoding quinolone-modifying enzymes, which are not frequently used in children but are widely used for empirical therapy of urinary tract infections in adults, and in practice patients improve. This resistance behaviour has become a health problem that is difficult to manage, as there are no other antibiotics for community use that allow empirical prescription as is usually applied, which we attribute to the frequent use of these drugs without periodic monitoring of sensitivity and resistance patterns that allow rotation with protocols in each region.Many studies on the subject have been carried out in Cuba and around the world, in most of them we find similarities with our results, others disagree, especially in relation to Ceftriaxone, as we have noticed that the oldest studies show very low levels of resistance, while the most recent ones, including ours, describe high patterns, from which we can deduce that there has been a progressive increase in bacterial resistance to this drug, which has been favoured by the use and abuse of the drug.

In industrialised countries, 53 per cent of paediatric UTI cases have been found to be resistant to Amoxicillin, one of the most commonly prescribed primary care antibiotics. Nearly a quarter of young patients in industrialised countries were resistant to the antibiotic Cotrimoxazole. Among children in developing countries, resistance was even higher. Nearly 80% of paediatric UTI cases in the poorest countries were resistant to Amoxicillin. More than a quarter were resistant to Ciprofloxacin (Cipro), and 17% to Nitrofurantoin (Macrobid). (22)

In the microbiology laboratory belonging to the Municipal Centre of Hygiene and Epidemiology, in Güines, in the period from 2003 to 2004, the strains showed sensitivity levels of over 90 % for Amikacin and between 85 % and 90 % for Ceftriaxone. Similar results were found in studies carried out in microbiology laboratories in Havana (1, 52, 61, 69).In the Mayabeque Provincial Microbiology Laboratory, in the municipality of San José de las Lajas, in the period between May and December 2012, in terms of the Antimicrobial susceptibility, it was observed that of the 86 strains of Escherichia coli against the 12 antimicrobial drugs, high levels of sensitivity were found for the urinary antiseptic Nitrofurantoin, with 90.6 %, Ceftriaxone showed a sensitivity below 50 %. However, Sulfaprim, Nalidixic acid and Ampicillin were the drugs that showed the lowest sensitivity to Escherichia coli strains, results that coincide with studies carried out in Holguín and Las Tunas (8,21, 58).Similar results have been found in investigations in children by Schito GC et al. 2003 in Italy, by Graninger W et al. 2003 in Austria, Anderson GG et al. 2004, and by Talan DA et al. 2004 in the United States. However, the results of these investigations disagree with those of an antimicrobial susceptibility surveillance project on Escherichia coli strains conducted in Europe (Pan-European ECOSENS), which found low levels of resistance to ampicillin and trimethoprim-sulfamethoxazole. (60)According to the Special Journal of Chemotherapy 2015, in a study carried out from 1 January 2011 to 31 December 2013, Escherichia coli strains isolated from urine cultures of patients from primary care in the Barbastro sector were studied, globally, there was an increase in the resistance of Escherichia coli isolates to all antimicrobials studied. However, resistance remained below 4% for Nitrofurantoin and below 10% for second and third generation cephalosporins. The highest levels of resistance (above 30%) were found in orally administered antibiotics frequently indicated for uncomplicated urinary tract infections: trimethoprim sulfamethoxazole, ciprofloxacin and ampicillin, in agreement with other international studies (65, 67, 70, 71, 72). (65, 67, 70, 71, 72).

The research carried out by the Laboratory of the National Secretariat for the Human Rights of Persons with Disabilities "Fernando de la Mora", in Paraguay, with respect to the resistance patterns for E. coli, showed that all strains were resistant to ampicillin 11/11 (100%), however, for Nitrofurantoin the sensitivity was 100% and for Ciprofloxacin 73%. (55)

Table IV: Infants with urinary tract infection. Distribution according to clinical forms of presentation. General Teaching Hospital "Comandante Pinares". San Cristóbal. 2017- 2019.

Clinical forms of presentation No. %

Typical	27	21.3
Asymptomatic	3	2.4
Feverish	28	22.0
Dystrophying	36	28.3
Fogging	8	6.3
Diarrhoea	20	15.7
Anaemic	1	0.8
Iteric	2	1.6
Pseudomeningeal	2	1.6
Toxic infectious	-	-
Total	127	100.0
Source: Medical records.		

Table IV analyses the clinical forms of presentation of urinary tract infections in the children studied, where we corroborate the dystrophic form as the most frequent with a total of 36 cases, for 28.3%, followed by the febrile and typical forms, with 22.0%

and 21.3% respectively. The literature on urinary tract infections describes that the most commonly identified symptoms on admission are fever, diarrhoea, straining, crying when urinating, insufficient weight gain, refusal of food, irritability, vomiting and jaundice, which explains that infants have atypical forms, and therefore an early diagnosis is necessary to avoid future complications (26).

When analysing the clinical forms of presentation in patients with a presumptive diagnosis of urinary sepsis, in the Hospital "General Milanés," of Bayamo, during 1999, acute febrile fever was observed as the most frequent with 38.7%, followed by gastroenteric fever with 37.1%. Similar results were obtained in the "Pedro Agustín Pérez" Paediatric Teaching Hospital in Guantánamo from January to December 2013, where the main reason for admission was fever with 222 cases for 58 %, followed by diarrhoea with 112 cases for 29.4 %, then lower urinary symptoms, such as sputum and symptoms of urinary incontinence. dysuric with 34 for 8.8% and insufficient weight gain or stationary weight with 8.8%.(57) However, in the Policlínico Comunitario Área Sur de Sancti Spíritus in the period from January 2003 to June 2004, the most frequent forms of presentation were urine staining the nappy, fever and stationary weight curve. According to Nelson, the most frequent symptom is fever, which was also the most frequently identified symptom in Colombia, Chile and Barcelona (49, 50, 73, 74, 75).

Table V: Infants with urinary tract infection. Distribution according to alterations in complementary examinations. General Teaching Hospital "Comandante Pinares". San Cristóbal. 2017- 2019.

Identified Alteration	No.	%
Anemia	34	26.8
Leukocytosis	52	40.9
Accelerated Erythrosedimentation	28	22.0
Leucocyturia	44	34.6
Ultrasonographic alterations	17	13.4
Source: Medical records.		

The tableV describes the main alterations identified in theexamscomplementary ests were carried out on the patients studied. Leukocyte counts were analysed and a predominance of patients with leukocytosis was observed: 52 (40.9%). This is due to the fact that the inflammatory response is activated by the physico-chemical contact between the surface of the invading germ and the cells of the bladder wall and leads to the release of chemotactic mediators that can also be released by the bacteria and produce the influx of polymorphonuclear cells that will cause the local inflammatory response and symptoms. This is not a study that defines urinary tract infection, but it can be stated that this alteration together with a suggestive clinical picture and the variations in the complementary examinations further support the diagnosis of urinary tract infection, which is in agreement with the literature reviewed (57, 61).

Of the total number of patients in the series, 34 (26.8%) had anaemia, which can be explained, firstly, by the physiological anaemia that exists in children under 1 year of age, which can be explained by This is aggravated by the fact that many of the micro-organisms that cause urinary tract infection, such as Escherichia coli and Proteus, are haemolysin producers; also, the production of aerobactins by these bacteria enables them to capture the iron necessary for their metabolism and multiplication, which reduces the iron available for haemoglobin production. These results coincide with those of other authors (57, 61).The erythrocyte sedimentation rate was accelerated in 28 (22.0%) of the cases studied. This corresponds to the findings of other authors, who state that there is accelerated erythrocyte sedimentation when pyelonephritis is present and, consequently, there is a greater likelihood of UTI appearing in this form the younger the age of the affected person. Although it does not offer a definitive diagnosis of the condition, it has a high percentage of positivity, so it is a means of confirmation when there is clinical suspicion of the disease and should not be overlooked in any of those affected. In this investigation, 44 (34.6%) of the patients studied had leucocyturia. The intensity of the urine leucocyte count is not as important as the presence of significant numbers, which is of great value in establishing a reasonable degree of immediate suspicion for urinary tract infection. These data are consistent with those reviewed in the international literature (57, 61).

On reviewing the abdominal and renal ultrasounds performed on these patients, we were able to identify anatomical alterations in 17 of them, representing 13.4% of the study sample, which were prominence of the pyramids and dilatation of the excretory system, mainly of the right kidney. In the investigation carried out at the Hospital Infantil Sur in Santiago de Cuba from January to December 2010, it was observed that most of the patients had anaemia, with lesser affectation of this parameter as age increased. Regarding blood leukocyte values, 37 patients had leukocytosis, which represented 57.8 % of the total, while 27 patients had normal figures, for 42.2

%. When correlating the erythrocyte sedimentation rate values, it was found that of the patients who underwent this complementary test, only 9 had normal results. Urine leukocyte counts were altered in all 64 patients, with varying intensity: slight leukocyturia in 51 cases (79.6 %), moderate in 8 cases (12.5 %) and severe in 5 cases (7.9 %). (61)In the Pediatric Teaching Hospital "Pedro Agustín Pérez" in Guantánamo, a study was carried out from January-December 2013, where it was found that cyturia was pathological in 283 children, 73.6 % of the total; in acute phase reactants, leukocytosis was present in 203 patients for 52.9 %, and accelerated erythrocyte sedimentation in 124 patients for 32.3 %. Nearly half of the patients studied were anaemic, 158 (41.1 %). Renal ultrasound performed in the acute phase of the disease was positive in 125 of the 384 patients, representing 32.5 % (57).

CONCLUSIONS

The behaviour of antimicrobial sensitivity and resistance to drugs of first choice was determined in infants in the Paediatric Department of the General Hospital "Comandante Pinares", where a 3:2 ratio of female to male was observed in urinary tract infections, except in the age group 1 to 3 months, where the male sex predominated, this age group also having a higher incidence. Escherichia coli was recognised as the most frequent cause of urinary tract infection, predominating in both sexes, followed by Enterobacter spp. and Proteus spp. 3rd generation cephalosporins showed high levels of resistance while Amikacin showed a low level, with Nitrofurantoin showing the highest sensitivity. The most frequent clinical forms of presentation were the dystrophic form, followed by the febrile and typical forms. A predominance of patients with leukocytosis and leukocyturia was observed.

RECOMMENDATIONS

Antimicrobial therapy should be carefully assessed before being initiated, taking into account the risk-benefit ratio in each case in order to avoid or reduce bacterial resistance. There should be well-established protocols in each unit, based on the well-documented microbiological map, for the correct use of antimicrobials, which will contribute to the reduction and control of bacterial resistance.

BIBLIOGRAPHICAL REFERENCES

1- Daggers Medel I., Monzote López A., Torres Amaro G., Hernández Robledo E. Bacterial etiology of urinary tract infection in children. Rev Cubana Med Gen Integr [Internet]. 2012 Dec [cited 2017 Feb 03] 28(4): 620-629. Available en: http://scielo.sld.cu/scielo.php?script=sci_arttext&pid=S0864-21252012000400006&lng=es.

2- González-Rodríguez JD, Rodríguez-Fernández LM. Urinary tract infection in childhood. Protoc diagn ter pediatr. 2014; 1:91-108.

3- Cross JR From la. Kidney and urinary tract infection. In: Gordillo PG, Exeni AR, De la Cruz JR. Nefrología Pediátrica.2ed.Madrid: Elsevier; 2010.p. 329-56.

4-Khan AU, Musharraf

A: Plasmid-mediated multiple antibiotic resistance in Proteus mirabilis isolated from patients with urinary tract infection. Med Sci Monit. 2014 Nov; 10(11): 598-602.

5- Valdevenito PS. Recurrent urinary tract infection in women. Rev CM Infect 2008; 25 (4): 268-276.

6-Bello-Fernandez ZL, Cozme-Rojas Y, Morales-Parada IC, Pacheco-Pérez Y, Rua-Del-Toro M. Antimicrobial resistance in pediatric patients with urinary tract infection. Revista Electrónica Dr. Zoilo E. Marinello Vidaurreta [journal on the Internet]. 2018 [cited 2019 Apr 11]; 43(2): [approx. 0 p.]. Available from: http://revzoilomarinello.sld.cu/index.php/zmv/article/view/1271

7-Alós JI. Resistance Bacterial resistance to antibiotics: a global crisis. Enferm Infecc Microbiol Clín [Internet]. dec. 2015 [cited 24 Jan 2016]; 33(10):692-699. Available from: http://www.sciencedirect.com/science/article/pii/S0213005X14003413

8-Espino Hernández M. Antimicrobial resistance: a global problem. Panorama. Cuba y Salud [Internet]. 2014 [cited 2019 Apr 11]; 6(1): [approx. 1 p.]. Available from: http://www.revpanorama.sld.cu/index.php/panorama/article/view/70

9-Rodríguez Rondón Y,Pantoja Prosper C, Beatón Matamoros O, Zúñiga Moro A, Rodríguez Sánchez VZ. Antimicrobial prescribing and its relationship with bacterial resistance in a municipal general hospital. MEDISAN [journal on the Internet]. 2017 [cited 2019 Apr 11]; 21(5): [approx. 0 p.]. Available from: http://medisan.sld.cu/index.php/san/article/view/1198

10- Goodman and Gilman. Pharmacological Basis of Therapeutics. In: Mandell GL, Petri WA, eds. Antimicrobial Drugs: Penicillins, Cephalosporins and other β-lactam antibiotics. 12ed. Madrid: McGraw Hill Interamericana; 2014.

11-Pino Muñoz M, Ojeda Pino B, Martínez Martínez M, Brougthon Ferriol J, González Ramírez G, Pina Rodríguez A. Behaviour of antimicrobial resistance in a closed neonatology department. MediCiego [Internet]. 2018 [cited 2019 Apr 11]; 19(1): [approx. 0 p.]. Available from: http://www.revmediciego.sld.cu/index.php/mediciego/article/view/200ç

12-Cruz Cruz Cruz EM. Antibiotics vs. bacterial resistance. Revista Electrónica Dr. Zoilo E. Marinello Vidaurreta [journal on the Internet]. 2015 [cited 2019 Apr 11]; 40(2): [approx. 0 p.]. Available from: http://revzoilomarinello.sld.cu/index.php/zmv/article/view/95

13-Drug resistance. Antimicrobial use [Internet]. Geneva: WHO; 2016 [cited 29 Apr 2016]. Available from: http://www.who.int/drugresistance/use/es/

14-Serra Valdés MÁ. Microbial resistance. A global health problem. Revista Habanera de Ciencias Médicas [journal on the Internet]. 2017 [cited]; 16(3): [310-311]. Available from: http://www.revhabanera.sld.cu/index.php/rhab/article/view/

15-https://boletinaldia.sld .cu/aldia/2017/02/28/publica-la-oms-lista-de-las-bacterias-para-las-que-se-necesitan- urgentemente-nuevos-antibioticos/

16-Rodrigo Gonzalo de Liria C, Méndez Hernández M, Azuara Robles M. Urinary tract infection. In: Protocols diagnóstico-terapéuticos de la AEP: Infectología pediátrica. [Monograph on the Internet]. Barcelona: Editorial ERGON; 2011[cited 6/2/2015]. Available from: https://www.aeped.es/sites/default/files/documentos/itu.pdf

17-Elías-Montes Y, Tamayo-Cordoví A, Ceballos-Yañez Y, Camejo-Serrano Y, Oduardo-Villa M. Risk factors for urinary tract infection in infants. General Paediatric Hospital Milanés. 2016. MULTIMED [journal on the Internet]. 2019 [cited 2019 Apr 9]; 23(2): [ca.13p.].Available from: http://www.revmultimed.sld.cu/index.php/mtm/article/view/1160

18-Mathijssen, A. J., Guzmán-Lastra, F., Kaiser, A., & Löwen, H. (2018). Nutrient Transport Driven by Microbial Active Carpets. Physical Review Letters, 121(24), 248101.https://boletinaldia.sld.cu/aldia/2018/12/26/fisicos-descubren-mecanismo-que-use-bacteria-to-become-resistant/

19https://boletinaldia.sld.cu/aldia/2017/03/30/investigan-la-aplicacion-de-bacteriofagos-as-alternativa-a-los- antibioticos/

20https://boletinaldia.sld.cu/aldia/2018/02/22/antibiotic-resistance-will-be-the-first-cause-of-death-in-2050/

21-Marrero Escalona JL, Leyva Toppes M, Castellanos Heredia JE. Urinary tract infection and antimicrobial resistance in the community. Rev Cubana Med Gen Integr. 2015 vol.31 (1)

22-https://boletinaldia.sld.cu/aldia/2016/03/24/antibiotic-resistance-is-common-in-children's-urinary-infections/

23-Ocen DG, CorridorJM. Urinary tract infection in paediatric patients in Hospital Bosa II level 2014. University of applied and environmental sciences. Faculty of Health Sciences/Medicine Program. Bogotá D.C. November. 2015

24-Pinzón-Fernández MV, Zúñiga-Cerón LF, Saavedra-Torres JS. Urinary tract infection in children, one of the most prevalent infectious diseases. Rev Fac Med 2018; 66(3):393-8.

25-Valdés Martin S.Urinary tract infection. In: Valdés Martin S, Gómez Vasallo A; Abreu Suarez G, Dávila A; Álvarez Arias CZ. Temas de Pediatría. 1 ed. Havana City: Ciencias Médicas 2016; p: 281-4.

26- Rubinstein A, Rahman G, Risso P. Fusion of the labia minora vulvae. Experience in a paediatric hospital. Arch Argent Pediatr 2018; 116(1):65-68.

27-Díaz M; Younen AA; Martínez H.Evaluation of the febrile newborn and prediction of urinary tract infection Rev Cubana Pediatr 1998; 70(4):170-75.

28-Gancedo García MC, Hernández Ganzedo MC. Acute and recurrent urinary tract infection. Pediatr Integral 2005; IX (5): 317-324.

29- Gauthier M, Chevalier I, Sterescu A, Bergeron S, Brunet S, Taddeo D. Treatment of urinary tract infections among young children with daily intravenous antibiotic therapy at a day treatment center. Pediatrics 2014; 114: 469-76.

30- Hoberman A, Charron M, Hickey R, Baskin M, Kearney D, Wald E. Imaging studies after a first febrile urinary tract infection in young children. N Engl J Med 2013; 348: 195-202.

31-Montini G, Rigon L, Zucchetta P, et al. Prophylaxis after first febrile urinary tract infection in children? A multicenter, randomized, controlled noninferiority trial. Pediatrics. 2015; 122(5):1064- 71.

32-Carbonell Noblet A, Rojas Turro Y. Study of antimicrobial drug use, prescription-indication. Rev. inf. cient. [Internet]. 2016 [cited 2019 Apr 11]; 95(3): [approx. 9 p.]. Available from: http://www.revinfcientifica.sld.cu/index.php/ric/article/view/127

33-Fariña N. Resistance bacterial infection: a global public health problem with a difficult solution. Mem. Inst. Inves. Sci. Salt [Internet]. 2016 Apr Accessed: 2017 Mar 17; 14(1): 04-05. Available from:

http://scielo.iics.una.py/scielo.php?script=sci_arttext&pid=S1812-95282016000100001&lng=en

34- World Health Organisation. Worldwide country situation analysis: response to antimicrobial resistance. World Health Organization. Geneva. [Internet]. April 2015 Accessed: 2017 Mar 20; Available from: http://www.who.int/drugresistance/e

35-Chavolla-Canal AJ,González-Mercado MG. Risk factors associated with urinary tract infection caused by superbugs. Rev Mex Urol. 2018; 78(6):425-33.

36-Ossa-Giraldo AC. Risk factors for multidrug-resistant Pseudomonas aeruginosa infection in a high complexity hospital. Rev Chil Infectol 2014; 31(4):393-399.

37- Marston HD, Dixon DM, Knisely JM, Palmore TN, Fauci AS. Antimicrobial resistance. Jama. [Internet]. 2016. Accessed: 2017 Mar 20; 316(11): 1193-1204. Available from: http://www.jama.jamanetwork.com/article.aspx?articleid

38- WHO. The WHO publishes the list of bacteria for which there is an emerging need for new antibiotics. [Internet]. 2017 Accessed: 17 March 2017; Available from: http://www.who.int/mediacentre/news/releases/2017/bacteria-antibiotics-needed/es/

39-WHO: What is the antimicrobial resistance? [Internet]. 2017. Accessed: 2017 Mar 18; Available from: Revista Habanera de Ciencias Médicas ISSN 1729-519X Page 416 http://www.who.int/features/qa/75/es/

40-Calderón Rojas G ,Aguilar Ulate L. Antimicrobial resistance: more resistant microorganisms and antibiotics with less activity. Rev Méd de Costa Rica y Centroa [Internet]. 2016. Accessed: 2017 Mar 19; 73(621):757-763. Available at: http://www.medigraphic.com/pdfs/revmedcoscen/rmc-2016/rmc164c.pdf

41- Becerra G,Plascencia A, Luévanos A, Domínguez M, Hernández I. Mechanism of antimicrobial resistance in bacteria. ENF INF MICROBIOL [Internet]. 2009. Accessed: 2017 Mar 19; 29 (2): 70-76. Available at: http://www.medigraphic.com/pdfs/micro/ei- 2009/ei092e.pdf.

42-Serra Valdés MA. The microbial resistance in the current context and the importance of knowledge and application in antimicrobial policy. Habanera Journal of Medical Sciences. 2017; 16(3): 17.

43-Rodríguez-Noriega E, León-Garnica G, Petersen-Morfín S, Pérez-Gómez H, González-Díaz E, Morfín- Otero R. The evolution of bacterial resistance in Mexico, 1973-2013. Biomédica: Revista Del Instituto Nacional De Salud [journal on the internet]. 2014 Apr [cited 2015 Feb 4]; 34(S1): 181-190. Available from: Medic Latina.

44-Serra Valdés MA. Antimicrobial policy. A pressing need in the face of today's growing microbial resistance. Rev haban cienc méd [Internet]. 2017 [Accessed:]; 16(4): 564-578. Available from:

http://www.revhabanera.sld.cu/index.php/rhab/article/view/2072

45-Alvarez Almanza D. Identification of extended-spectrum beta-lactamases in enterobacteria. Revista Habanera de Ciencias Médicas [journal on the Internet].2018 [Cited 2019 Apr 11]; 9(4): [approx.0p.].Available at:

http://www.revhabanera.sld.cu/index.php/rhab/article/view/1716

46-Hernández Martínez EM, Marín Conde Y, Carrazana García D, Vales Almodóva M, Ramos Villanueva Y. Consumption and resistance to antibacterials in a second level hospital. Medicentro Electrónica [Internet]. 2016 Dec; 20(4): 268-277. [Accessed: 2017 Jun 22]. Available at:

http://scielo.sld.cu/scielo.php?script=sci_arttext&pid=S1029-30432016000400004&lng=es

47-Ruvinsky S, Monaco A, Pérez G, Taicz M, Inda L, Epelbaum C, et al. Effectiveness of a programme to improve antibiotic use in children admitted to a tertiary care paediatric hospital in Argentina.Arch. argent. pediatr. [Internet]. 2014 Apr; 112(2): 124-

131.[Accessed:2017Jun22].Available en:

http://www.scielo.org.ar/scielo.php?script=sci_arttext&pid=S0325-00752014000200004&lng=es

48-Fernandez-Ruiz D , Quiros-Enríquez M, Cuevas-Pérez O, Rodríguez-Herrera E, Padilla-Labrado M. Advanced course on antimicrobial selection and management in respiratory and urinary tract infections. Medisur [journal on the Internet]. 2015 [cited 2019 Apr 11]; 13.(2):[approx.6p.]. Available at:

http://www.medisur.sld.cu/index.php/medisur/article/view/2913

49-Malo Rodríguez G , Echeverry J, Iragorri S, Gastelbondo R. Clinical practice guidelines. Urinary tract infection in children under 2 years of age. Rev Col Ped [Internet]. 2010 [cited5Nov2016]; 36(3):9- 13.Available from:

https://encolombia.com/medicina/revistas-medicas/pediatria/vp- 363/pedi36301-sociedadguia/

50- Espinosa RL. Urinary tract infection. In: Garcías Nieto V, Santos F. Nefrología Pediátrica.2ed. Spain: Aula Méd; 2012.p.205-16.

51-Córdoba L, Machado O, Valdés F, Dueñas E, Amador M, Duyos H, et al. Normas de Pediatría. 4ed. Havana: Editorial Ciencias Médicas; 2013.p.431-37

52- Díaz Álvarez M, Cárdenas González L. Aseptic meningitis concurrent with urinary tract infection in newborns. Rev Cubana Ped [Internet]. 2011 [cited 22 Dec 2016]; 83(1):130-141. ISSN 1028-9933 212 Available at: http://scieloprueba.sld.cu/pdf/ped/v83n2/ped02211.pdf

53-Hay AD, Birnie K, Busby J, Delaney B, Downing H, Dudley J, et al. The Diagnosis of Urinary Tract infection in Young children (DUTY): a diagnostic prospective observational study to derive and validate a clinical algorithm for the diagnosis of urinary tract infection in children presenting to primary care with an acute illness. Health Technol Assess. 2016; 20(51):1-294. Available at: http://scielo.sld.cu/pdf/ped/v90n2/ped06218.pdf

54-Encalada F . Á Luque M. V. M. M., Jaramillo M. E. C., & Chica H. A. P. Renal complications in preschool paediatric patients with a history of urinary tract infection. RECIMUNDO: Scientific Journal of Research and Knowledge. 2018; 2(2): 394-405

55-Molin C, Del Valle E, González L, Figueredo L. Urinary tract infections in children with neurogenic bladder and patterns of resistance to the most frequent uropathogens. Mem. Inst. Investig. Sci. Health. 2018; 16(3): 44-50

56-Lombardo-Aburto E . Paediatric approach to urinary tract infections. Acta Pediatr Mex. 2018; 39(1):85-90.

57-Delgado Velázquez R, Benítez Fuentes M, Hernández Cardosa M. Urinary tract infection in infants. Rev. inf. cient. [Internet]. 2017 [cited 2019 Apr 11]; 96(2): [approx. 7 p.]. Available from: http://www.revinfcientifica.sld.cu/index.php/ric/article/view/13.

58- Towers Fuentes Generoso, Brito Herrera Belkis, Barbier Rubiera Amarilys. Behaviour of the urinary tract infection and antimicrobial susceptibility of the most frequent bacteria. Rev Cubana Med Gen Integr [Internet]. 2014 Dec [cited 2019 Apr 01]; 30(4): 416-425. Availableat:http://scielo.sld.cu/scielo.php?script=sci_arttext&pid=S0864-21252014000400003&lng=es.

59-Cabrera NE, Cleger FM, Martínez HM, Gulgar WV, Otamendi FC, Velázquez LX, et al. Uso de Antimicrobianos en infección del tracto urinario [Thesis]. Guantánamo: Hospital Pediátrico Docente "Pedro Agustín Pérez"; 2007.

60-Díaz Rigau Leonor,Cabrera Rodríguez Luis Enrique, Fernández Núñez Tania, González Febles Ortelio, Carrasco Guzmán Miguel, Bravo Laura. Bacterial aetiology of urinary tract infection and antimicrobial susceptibility in Escherichia coli strains. Rev Cubana Pediatr [Internet]. 2006 Sep [cited 2017 Feb 03]; 78(3):Available en: http://scielo.sld.cu/scielo.php?script=sci_arttext&pid=S0034-

7531200600030000S&lng=es

61- Collado Garcia Oscar, Barreto Rodríguez Herlinda, Rodríguez Torrens Herlinda, Barreto Argilagos Guillermo, Abreu Guirado Orlando. Bacterial species associated with urinary tract infections. AMC [Internet]. 2017 Aug [cited 2019 Apr 01]; 21(4): 479-486. Available At: http://scielo.sld.cu/scielo.php?script=sci_arttext&pid=S1025-02552017000400006&lng=es

62-Chavez IslandMargarita Isabel, Rodríguez Hechavarría Félix, Chávez Solís Leonardo F. Laboratory diagnosis in patients admitted for urinary tract infection in a paediatric hospital. MEDISAN [Internet]. 2012 Jan [cited 2017 Feb 10]; 16(1): 56-61. Available from: http://scielo.sld.cu/scielo.php?script=sci_arttext&pid=S1029-30192012000100008&lng=en.

63-Díaz L, Cabrera L, Fernández T, González O, Carrasco M, Bravo L. Bacterial etiology of urinary tract infection and antimicrobial susceptibility in Escherichia coli strains. Rev Cubana Pediatr. 2006 [accessed 11 Jan 2013]; 78 (3):42-45. Available at: http://scielo.sld.cu/scielo.php?script=sci_serial&

64-Alvarado Sosa J,Mejía Villatoro C. Bacterial Resistance in Urinary Tract Infections of Urinary Tract Origin. Community. [Online] 2016 [Accessed 2018 March 21]; 20 (1): p.24. Available from:http://asomigua.org/wp-content/uploads/2016/08/articulo-3.pdf

65-Guerra Lloacana DD. Bacterial resistance to fluoroquinolones in outpatients with urinary tract infections treated at the Hospital Enrique Garcés in the period January-August 2017. Thesis work prior to obtaining the degree of Licenciado en Laboratorio Clínico e Histotecnológico. Career of Clinical and Histotechnological Laboratory. Quito: UCE. 2018. 67 p.

66-https://seq.es/seq/02 14-3429/29/3/moya19apr2016.pdf

67-Castrillón Spitia JD, Machado-Alba JE, Gómez Idarraga S, Gómez Gutiérrez M, Remolina León N, Ríos Gallego JJ. Etiology and antimicrobial resistance profile in patients with urinary tract infection. Infect [Internet]. 2019 Jan [cited 2019 Apr 09]; 23(1): 45-51. Available from: http://www.scielo.org.co/scielo.php?script=sci_arttext&pid=S0123-93922019000100045&lng=en. http://dx.doi.org/10.22354/in.v23i1.755.

68-López C, Reyes G, Gallegos B, Reyes D, Reyes K. Urinary bacteriology in children with disabilities. Enf.Inf.Microbiol. 2014; 34 (1):26-30.)

69- Suarez Trueba B, Milián Samper Y, Espinosa Rivera F, Hart Casares M, Llanes

Rodríguez N, Martínez Batista ML. Antimicrobial susceptibility antimicrobial susceptibility y mechanisms of resistance of Escherichia coli isolated from urine cultures in a tertiary hospital. Rev cubana med [Internet]. 2014 Mar [cited 2019 Apr 01]; 53(1): 3-13. Available from: http://scielo.sld.cu/scielo.php?script=sci_arttext&pid=S0034-75232014000100002&lng=en.

70-Beltrán A, Cortez A, López C. Evaluation of antibiotic resistance of Escherichia coli in community-acquired urinary tract infections in the health sector of Barbastro. Rev Esp Quimioter. 2015

71-Orrego-Marín CP,Henao-Mejía CP, Cardona-Arias JA. Prevalence of urinary tract infection, uropathogens and antimicrobial susceptibility profile. Acta Médica Colombiana. 2014; 39(4):353.

72-Valverde RA, Idrogo JJ, Significance FR, Alva R. Community-acquired upper urinary tract infection with E. coli resistant to ciprofloxacin: associated characteristics in patients from a national hospital in Peru. An Fac med. 2015; 76(4):385-91

73-Nelson Waldo E. Urinary tract infection. In: Behrman R, Kliegman R, Arvin Ann M. Treatise on Paediatrics. 19ed. v.II. Havana: Editorial Ciencias Médicas; 2011.p.2005-11.

74-Moriyón JC, Petit N,Coronel V, Ariza M, Arias A, Orta N. Urinary tract infection in paediatrics: definition, epidemiology, pathogenesis, diagnosis. Arch Ven Puer Ped [Internet].2011 [cited 3 Mar2016]; 74(1): [approx. 13 p.]. Available en: http://www.scielo.org.ve/scielo.php?script=sci_arttext&pid=S0004-06492011000100006

75- Cavagnaro F. Urinary tract infection in paediatrics: controversies. Rev Chilena Infectol [Internet]. 2012 [cited 22 Dec 2016]; 29(4): 427- 433 [cited10 Nov2016]. Available from: http://www.scielo.cl/pdf/rci/v29n4/art10.pdf

ANNEXES

Annex 1. Informed consent. Paediatric Department

General Teaching Hospital "Comandante Pinares".

Consent of parents, relatives or guardians of the child to participate in the research:
Antimicrobial resistance to drugs of choice in infants with urinary tract infections.
Hospital "Comandante Pinares", 2017-2019.

I have read and understood the information given to me about the research. I have
been able to ask all the questions that concerned me about the research, obtaining
satisfactory answers. I have received sufficient information about the work,
understanding that my participation is voluntary and that I can withdraw from it
whenever I wish, without having to give explanations and without this having
repercussions on my child's medical care.

I have been informed that the investigator will ensure that this study is conducted in
accordance with the provisions in which the research is carried out, which afford
maximum protection to the patient.

In view of the above, I hereby give my consent to be included in the children's
research.

Signature of the patient or authorised relative:
Name and signature of the physician:

Behaviour of antimicrobial sensitivity and resistance to drugs of first choice in infants in the Paediatric Department of the General Hospital "Comandante Pinares".

Questionnaire:

1.Name and surname:

2.Age:

1 - 3 months

4- 6 months

7- 9 months

10- 12 months

3.Sex:

Male Female

4.Clinical form of presentation:

Typical

Asymptomatic

Febrile

Dystrophic

Emetising

Diarrhoea

Anaemic

Icteric

Pseudomeningeal

Toxic-infectious

5.Complementary examinations:

Hb:NormalDecreased

Leukogram:Normal Elevated

Erythrocyte sedimentation: Normal Accelerated

Cyturia: Positive Negative

Renal ultrasound: Normal Altered

Alteration:

6. Positive urine cultures:Yes:No

Isolated germ:

7. Antibiogram:

Antibiotic

Sensitive

Resistant

Ceftriaxone

Cefotaxime

Amikacin

Nitrofurantoin

Cotrimoxazole

Ciprofloxacin

Nalidixic acid

Cephalexin

Amoxicillin

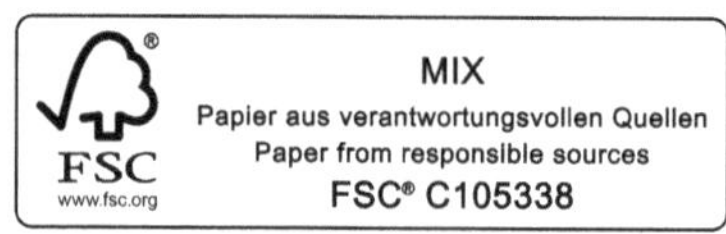

Printed by Books on Demand GmbH, Norderstedt / Germany